WHAT

TO KNOW AS A

FIRST TIME

MOM

: A COMPREHENSIVE

GUIDE FOR

FIRST TIME

MOMS

By

Laura Warsh

Table of Contents

Eat Nutritious Foods:

Gentle Exercise

Seek Help When Needed:

Practice Self-Care:

Connect with Other Moms:

CHAPTER 4

Understanding Your Baby's Development and Milestones

Physical development

Cognitive development:

Language development:

Social and emotional development:

Establishing a support system and seeking help when needed are crucial for new mothers. Here are some tips on how to do it

Talk to your healthcare provider:

Consider hiring a postpartum doula:

Take advantage of resources in your community

Prioritize self-care:

Take care of yourself

Don't stress about it:

Practical Advice and Strategies for Navigating the Transition to Motherhood and Adjusting to the Demands and Joys of Caring for a Newborn

Take care of yourself:

Accept help:

Learn to trust your instincts:

Prioritize sleep:

Stay connected

Embrace flexibility

TAKE TIME FOR YOUR PARTNER

Seek professional help when needed

CONCLUSION

PREFACE

Becoming a mother for the first time is an exhilarating and challenging experience. There are so many new things to learn, decisions to make, and emotions to navigate. As a first-time mom, you may feel overwhelmed and unsure of what to expect.

This book is designed to help you navigate this exciting but sometimes overwhelming journey of motherhood. It provides practical advice, tips, and insights to help you prepare for the physical and emotional changes of pregnancy, childbirth, and early parenting.

In this book, you will learn about the different stages of pregnancy and what to expect during each trimester. You will discover the various childbirth options available to you and how to prepare for the delivery of your baby. You will also learn about the different methods of infant feeding, how to care for a newborn, and how to cope with the challenges of early parenthood.

The information in this book is based on the latest research and the experiences of other first-time moms. It covers everything from preconception planning to postpartum recovery, and is designed to help you feel confident and empowered as you embark on this new journey.

Whether you are feeling excited, anxious, or a combination of both, this book is here to support you. It is a comprehensive guide that will provide you with the information and resources you need to make informed decisions and navigate the ups and downs of motherhood.

So take a deep breath, relax, and let's get started on this exciting new adventure together.

INTRODUCTION

Becoming a first-time mom is a life-changing experience that can be both exhilarating and overwhelming. As you embark on this new journey, you may have countless questions and concerns about pregnancy, childbirth, and parenting. You may feel excited and anxious at the same time, wondering if you are ready for the challenges and joys that lie ahead.

This book, "What to Know as a First Time Mom," is designed to provide you with the essential information and guidance you need to navigate this exciting but uncertain time. Whether you are in the early stages of pregnancy or have just welcomed your little one into the world, this book will offer practical tips and advice to help you feel more confident and prepared for the journey ahead.

From understanding the physical and emotional changes of pregnancy to caring for a newborn, this book will cover a wide range of topics to help you make informed decisions and feel empowered as a first-time mom. You will learn about the various childbirth options, ways to stay healthy during pregnancy, and tips for postpartum recovery. Additionally, you will discover how to establish a support system, balance your new role with other responsibilities, and address common concerns and challenges that arise in early motherhood.

Whether you are a first-time mom-to-be or a new mom navigating the early stages of parenting, this book is your ultimate guide to feeling confident, empowered, and prepared for the journey ahead. So let's get started on this exciting and life-changing adventure together!

CHAPTER 1

Understanding the Physical and Emotional Changes that Occur During Pregnancy

Pregnancy is an exciting and transformative time in a woman's life, but it can also bring about significant physical and emotional changes. As a first-time mom, it's important to understand these changes and how they may affect your body and overall well-being.

Physical Changes

During pregnancy, your body goes through many changes as it adapts to support the growing life inside you. Some of the most notable physical changes include:

Weight gain: You may gain between 25-35 pounds during pregnancy, with most of the weight being gained in the second and third trimesters.

Hormonal changes: Your body produces higher levels of hormones such as estrogen and progesterone, which can lead to symptoms like nausea, fatigue, and mood swings.

Changes in your breasts: As your body prepares for breastfeeding, your breasts may become sore, swollen, and tender.

Changes in your skin: Many women experience changes in their skin during pregnancy, including stretch marks, acne, and darkening of the skin around the nipples and genitals.

Changes in your digestive system: Hormonal changes can slow down digestion, leading to constipation and heartburn.

Emotional Changes

In addition to the physical changes, pregnancy can also bring about a range of emotional changes. Some common emotional changes include:

Mood swings: Hormonal changes can cause mood swings, leading to feelings of happiness, anxiety, or sadness.

Anxiety and worry: It's normal to feel anxious or worried about the health of your baby and the upcoming birth.

Excitement: Many women feel a sense of excitement and anticipation as they prepare to become a mother.

Fatigue: It's common to feel tired during pregnancy, particularly in the first and third trimesters.

Bonding with your baby: As you feel your baby move and grow inside you, you may experience a strong bond and connection with your child.

It's important to remember that every woman's experience of pregnancy is unique, and that the physical and emotional changes you experience may differ from those of other women. However, by understanding the common changes that occur during pregnancy, you can better prepare for and cope with this transformative time in your life.

CHAPTER 2

Preparing for Childbirth

One of the most important aspects of becoming a first-time mom is preparing for childbirth. This can be a daunting and overwhelming process, but with the right information and support, you can feel more confident and empowered throughout your pregnancy and delivery. In this chapter, we'll discuss some key considerations for preparing for childbirth, including choosing a birth plan and considering pain management options.

Choosing a Birth Plan

One of the first decisions you'll need to make when preparing for childbirth is choosing a birth plan. A birth plan is a written document that outlines your preferences for how you'd like your labor and delivery to proceed. This can include things like:

Where you want to give birth (e.g. hospital, birthing center, at home)

Who you want to be present during labor and delivery

Your preferences for pain management options

Your preferences for fetal monitoring and interventions

Your preferences for delivery positions

Your preferences for postpartum care

It's important to keep in mind that a birth plan is not set in stone and may need to be adjusted based on your individual circumstances and medical needs. However, having a birth plan can help you communicate your wishes with your healthcare provider and ensure that you're involved in the decision-making process.

Considering Pain Management Options

Another important consideration when preparing for childbirth is deciding on pain management options. While childbirth can be a natural and empowering experience, it can also be quite painful. There are a variety of pain management options available, ranging from non-medical techniques to medication and anesthesia. Some common options include:

Breathing techniques and relaxation exercises

Hydrotherapy (e.g. using a birthing pool)

Massage and other bodywork

Nitrous oxide (laughing gas)

Epidural anesthesia

It's important to do your research and discuss your options with your healthcare provider to determine the best pain management plan for your individual needs and preferences.

By choosing a birth plan and considering pain management options, you can feel more prepared and empowered as you approach childbirth. Remember, every woman's experience is unique, and there's no one "right" way to give birth. The most important thing is to stay informed, communicate with your healthcare provider, and trust in your own instincts and abilities.

Tips for a Healthy Pregnancy

As a first time mom, you're probably eager to do everything you can to ensure a healthy pregnancy. Here are some tips to help you along the way:

Proper Nutrition: Eating a balanced and healthy diet is crucial during pregnancy. Make sure to include plenty of fruits, vegetables, lean protein, and whole grains in your meals. Avoid processed and junk food, as well as foods that are high in sugar or caffeine. Stay hydrated by drinking plenty of water throughout the day.

Prenatal Vitamins: Your doctor will likely recommend taking prenatal vitamins during pregnancy. These supplements contain important nutrients like folic acid, iron, and calcium that are essential for your baby's growth and development.

Exercise: Regular exercise can help you maintain a healthy weight, reduce your risk of gestational diabetes, and improve your overall wellbeing. Aim to get at least 30 minutes of moderate exercise most days of the week, such as walking, swimming, or prenatal yoga. Be sure to consult with your doctor before starting any new exercise program.

Rest: Getting enough rest is important during pregnancy. Try to get 7-8 hours of sleep each night and take breaks during the day if you're feeling tired.

Remember, every pregnancy is different and it's important to listen to your body and follow your doctor's advice. By taking care of yourself during pregnancy, you're setting the foundation for a healthy and happy pregnancy and baby Caring for a newborn, including feeding, diapering, and bathing.

CHAPTER 3

Caring for Your Newborn

One of the biggest adjustments you'll make as a first-time mom is learning how to care for your newborn. In this chapter, we'll cover some of the essential tasks you'll need to master, including feeding, diapering, and bathing.

Feeding: Breastfeeding is the recommended way to feed your baby, but it can take time to get the hang of it. Don't hesitate to ask for help from a lactation consultant or other experienced moms. If you're unable to breastfeed, formula is a safe and healthy alternative.

Diapering: Your baby will go through a lot of diapers in the first few weeks of life. Be prepared with plenty of diapers, wipes, and diaper cream. Make sure to change your baby's diaper frequently to prevent diaper rash and infections.

Bathing: Newborns don't need to be bathed every day, but you should clean their diaper area and face regularly. Use a mild soap and warm water, and be careful not to get water in your baby's ears or eyes.

By mastering these basic skills, you'll be well on your way to providing the best possible care for your little one.

Navigating Postpartum Recovery and Self-Care

Postpartum recovery and self-care are important aspects of a new mother's experience. After giving birth, your body needs time to heal, and you may also be adjusting to the physical, emotional, and lifestyle changes that come with motherhood.

Here are some tips for navigating postpartum recovery and self-care;

Prioritize Rest: It's essential to get enough rest during the early weeks and months after childbirth. Make sure you're taking time to rest whenever possible and asking for help from friends or family members if needed. Try to nap when your baby is sleeping, and don't worry about household chores or other tasks.

Eat Nutritious Foods: Your body needs nourishing foods to recover from childbirth and produce breast milk. Focus on eating a balanced diet with plenty of fruits, vegetables, whole grains, and lean proteins. Stay hydrated by drinking plenty of water.

Gentle Exercise: While it's important to rest, light exercise can help promote healing and reduce stress. Ask your healthcare provider about safe exercise options, such as walking or gentle yoga, and start slowly.

Seek Help When Needed: It's common to experience some physical and emotional challenges after childbirth. If you're feeling overwhelmed, anxious, or depressed, don't hesitate to seek help from your healthcare provider or a mental health professional. Postpartum depression is a serious condition that requires treatment.

Practice Self-Care: Self-care is essential for your physical and emotional well-being. Take time for yourself to do things you enjoy, such as reading, taking a bath, or going for a walk. Ask your partner or a trusted friend or family member to watch your baby while you take some time for yourself.

Connect with Other Moms: Joining a new mom's group or attending a breastfeeding support group can be a great way to connect with other moms who are going through similar experiences. You can share advice, offer support, and build friendships.

In summary, navigating postpartum recovery and self-care is an important aspect of the new mother's experience. By prioritizing rest, eating nutritious foods, getting gentle exercise, seeking help when needed, practicing self-care, and connecting with other moms, you can support your physical and emotional well-being during this transition.

CHAPTER 4

Understanding Your Baby's Development and Milestones

Understanding your baby's development and milestones is an essential part of the journey of motherhood. As a first-time mom, it can be overwhelming to figure out what is "normal" and what to expect as your baby grows and develops. That's why a section on this topic is crucial in a book titled "Things to Know as a First-Time Mom."

Babies develop at their own pace, and there is a wide range of what is considered "normal" when it comes to hitting developmental milestones. However, there are some general patterns that can help you understand what to expect as your baby grows.

The first year of your baby's life is a time of incredible growth and development. During this time, your baby will go from a helpless newborn who is entirely dependent on you to a mobile, curious, and increasingly independent little person.

Some of the key milestones you can expect to see during your baby's first year include:

Physical development: Your baby will learn to lift their head, roll over, sit up, crawl, and eventually walk.

Cognitive development: Your baby will begin to understand cause and effect, recognize familiar faces and objects, and develop problem-solving skills.

Language development: Your baby will start to make sounds, babble, and eventually say their first words.

Social and emotional development: Your baby will learn to bond with you and other caregivers, develop a sense of trust, and show a range of emotions, from joy to frustration.

As a first-time mom, it can be helpful to track your baby's milestones and talk to your pediatrician if you have any concerns. However, it's important to remember that all babies develop at their own pace, and some may hit milestones earlier or later than others. The most important thing is to provide a safe, nurturing environment for your baby and to enjoy the journey of watching them grow and develop.

Establishing a support system and seeking help when needed are crucial for new mothers. Here are some tips on how to do it

Reach out to family and friends: Don't hesitate to ask for help from those closest to you, whether it's a family member or a close friend. Let them know that you appreciate their support, and be specific about what kind of help you need. It can be anything from bringing over a meal to watching the baby while you take a nap.

Join a mom's group: Consider joining a mom's group in your area or an online support group. These groups can provide you with a sense of community and a place to connect with other moms who are going through similar experiences.

Talk to your healthcare provider: Your healthcare provider can be a great resource for information and support. Don't be afraid to ask questions or express your concerns

Consider hiring a postpartum doula: A postpartum doula is a trained professional who provides support to new mothers and their families during the postpartum period. They can help with things like breastfeeding, newborn care, and household tasks.

Take advantage of resources in your community: There may be local resources available to new mothers, such as support groups, parenting classes, and lactation consultants. Research what's available in your area and take advantage of these resources.

Prioritize self-care: Remember that taking care of yourself is just as important as taking care of your baby. Don't be afraid to ask for help if you need it, and make time for activities that help you recharge and feel good.

By establishing a support system and seeking help when needed, you can reduce stress and feel more confident in your role as a new mother. Don't be afraid to reach out and ask for help when you need it, as it's a sign of strength, not weakness.

CHAPTER 5

Balancing Motherhood with Other Responsibilities, such as Work and Relationships

One of the biggest challenges for new mothers is balancing the demands of motherhood with other responsibilities, such as work and relationships. This can be especially challenging for first-time moms who are still adjusting to the demands of caring for a newborn. In this chapter, we will explore some strategies for balancing motherhood with work and relationships.

First and foremost, it's important to recognize that being a new mother is a full-time job in itself. The demands of caring for a newborn can be overwhelming, and it's important to give yourself permission to prioritize your baby's needs and your own needs for rest and recovery. This may mean taking time off from work or scaling back your work hours temporarily, and communicating with your partner, friends, and family about your needs for support.

When it comes to balancing work and motherhood, there are several strategies that can help. One is to plan ahead and be proactive about managing your time. This may mean scheduling work tasks around your baby's nap schedule, or negotiating with your employer for more flexible work hours or the ability to work from home. Many companies now offer maternity leave and flexible work arrangements, so it's worth exploring your options and advocating for what you need.

Another important strategy is to seek out support and resources. This may include finding a trusted childcare provider or a supportive community of other working moms. Many workplaces offer resources such as lactation rooms and breastfeeding support, which can help make the transition back to work smoother. It's also important to be realistic about what you can and can't do, and to seek help when you need it. Don't be afraid to ask your partner, friends, or family members for help with childcare or household tasks.

When it comes to balancing motherhood with relationships, there are several things to keep in mind. One is to communicate openly and honestly with your partner about your needs and expectations. This may mean setting boundaries around work and household tasks, or finding ways to carve out quality time for each other despite the demands of parenthood.

It's also important to prioritize self-care and to make time for your own interests and hobbies. This may mean taking a yoga class, going for a run, or simply carving out time for a relaxing bath or a good book. Taking care of your own needs will help you feel more energized and fulfilled, and will ultimately benefit your relationships with others.

Finally, don't forget to celebrate the joys of motherhood and to savor the moments with your baby. It's easy to get caught up in the demands of work and relationships, but it's important to take time to appreciate the beauty and wonder of your new role as a mother. Whether it's watching your baby take his or her first steps or simply cuddling together on the couch, these moments are precious and fleeting.

Balancing motherhood with other responsibilities can be challenging, but it's not impossible. By prioritizing self-care, seeking out support and resources, and communicating openly with your partner and others, you can find a balance that works for you and your family. Remember to be kind to yourself, and to enjoy the many rewards that come with being a first-time mom.

Addressing common concerns and challenges faced by new mothers,

Sleep Deprivation: Newborns need to be fed every few hours, which can make it difficult for new moms to get a good night's sleep. To cope with sleep deprivation, it's important to prioritize rest when you can. Try to nap when your baby naps, accept help from family and friends, and consider hiring a babysitter or postpartum doula to give you a break. Additionally, establishing a consistent bedtime routine for your baby can help them sleep better, which can lead to more sleep for you.

Postpartum Depression: Many new moms experience feelings of sadness, anxiety, and fatigue after giving birth. This is known as postpartum depression (PPD) and can be caused by a combination of hormonal changes, sleep deprivation, and the stress of caring for a new baby. If you suspect you may have PPD, it's important to seek help from a healthcare provider.

Treatment may include therapy, medication, or both.

Breastfeeding Challenges: Breastfeeding can be difficult for some new moms, and it's common to experience challenges such as sore nipples, difficulty latching, and low milk supply. To overcome these challenges, seek support from a lactation consultant or breastfeeding support group. Additionally, be patient with yourself and your baby - it may take time to establish a successful breastfeeding routine.

Postpartum Body Changes: Your body goes through many changes during and after pregnancy, and it can be challenging to adjust to your new body. Be kind to yourself and remember that it takes time to recover and regain strength. Consider taking up gentle exercise such as yoga or walking, and focus on eating a healthy, balanced diet.

Balancing Responsibilities: Many new moms struggle with balancing the demands of motherhood with other responsibilities such as work and relationships. It's important to prioritize self-care and set realistic expectations for yourself. Consider delegating tasks or seeking help from family and friends, and try to establish a routine that works for you and your family.

By addressing these common concerns and challenges, the book "Things to Know as a First Time Mom" can provide new mothers with practical advice and strategies for navigating the ups and downs of motherhood.

CHAPTER 6

Maximizing Sleep as a First-Time Mom

Sleep when the baby sleeps: This may be easier said than done, but taking naps when your baby is sleeping can help you get the rest you need.

Accept help: Don't be afraid to ask for help from your partner, family members, or friends. Having someone else take care of the baby for a few hours can give you a much-needed break.

Create a sleep-conducive environment: Make sure your bedroom is quiet, dark, and cool. Use blackout curtains, earplugs, and a white noise machine if necessary.

Develop a bedtime routine: Establish a calming bedtime routine for yourself, such as taking a warm bath or reading a book, to help you relax and prepare for sleep.

Prioritize sleep: Remember that getting enough sleep is essential for your health and well-being, as well as for your ability to care for your baby. Make sleep a priority and try to adjust your schedule accordingly.

Avoid caffeine and alcohol: Both caffeine and alcohol can interfere with sleep, so it's best to avoid them or consume them in moderation.

Consider co-sleeping: If you feel comfortable and it's safe for you and your baby, co-sleeping can help you get more sleep and make nighttime feedings easier.

Take care of yourself: Remember to take care of yourself by eating well, staying hydrated, and getting some exercise. A healthy lifestyle can help you sleep better.

Don't stress about it: Finally, try not to stress too much about getting enough sleep. It's normal to experience sleep disruptions as a new mom, and it will get easier over time. Just do your best to take care of yourself and your baby, and the rest will fall into place.

Practical Advice and Strategies for Navigating the Transition to Motherhood and Adjusting to the Demands and Joys of Caring for a Newborn

Take care of yourself: It's easy to get caught up in the demands of caring for a newborn, but it's important to prioritize your own self-care as well. Make sure to get plenty of rest, eat nutritious foods, and take time for activities that make you happy and relaxed, such as taking a warm bath or going for a walk.

Accept help: Don't be afraid to accept help from friends, family, or professionals. Whether it's someone bringing you a meal, helping with laundry, or hiring a postpartum doula, accepting help can give you much-needed support and relief.

Learn to trust your instincts: You may feel overwhelmed or unsure of yourself as a new mom, but remember that you know your baby best. Trust your instincts when it comes to feeding, comforting, and caring for your newborn.

Prioritize sleep: Sleep deprivation is a common challenge for new moms, but getting enough rest is essential for your health and well-being. Consider establishing a bedtime routine for your baby, and take naps when you can.

Stay connected: Isolation can be a problem for new moms, but staying connected with other parents or support groups can help you feel less alone. Consider joining a local mom's group or connecting with other parents online.

Embrace flexibility: Parenting can be unpredictable, and things don't always go according to plan. Embrace flexibility and be willing to adjust your expectations and plans as needed.

Take time for your partner: The transition to parenthood can be a strain on your relationship, so make sure to prioritize time with your partner. Consider scheduling regular date nights or finding other ways to reconnect and communicate.

Seek professional help when needed: If you're struggling with postpartum depression or anxiety, or if you have concerns about your baby's health or development, don't hesitate to seek professional help. Your doctor or a mental health professional can provide valuable support and resources.

Overall, the transition to motherhood can be challenging, but with the right support, strategies, and mindset, you can navigate this exciting and rewarding journey.

CONCLUSION

Becoming a first-time mom is an exciting and rewarding journey, but it can also be overwhelming and challenging. "What to Know as a First-Time Mom" is a comprehensive guide that covers everything you need to know to make this transition as smooth as possible. From pregnancy to early parenting, this book provides practical advice, tips, and strategies to help you navigate this new chapter in your life with confidence and ease. Whether you are feeling anxious or excited about motherhood, this book is here to support you every step of the way. Remember, being a mom is not easy, but with the right tools and information, you can be the best mom you can be for your little one.